# Clinical Governance:
## one year on

### *Edited by Alastair D Scotland*

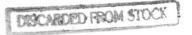

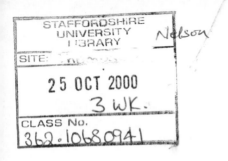
Quay Books Division, Mark Allen Publishing Ltd,
Jesses Farm, Snow Hill, Dinton, Salisbury, Wilts, SP3 5HN

Bristish library Cataloguing-in-Publication Data
A catalogue record is available for this book

© Mark Allen Publishing Ltd 2000
ISBN 1 85642 185 6

Printed in the UK by The Cromwell Press, Trowbridge, Wilts

# Contents

# Preface
# Clinical Governance: one year on

*Alastair D Scotland FRCS FRCP FFPHM*

Clinical governance as a term has been coined as a central plank of the present government's strategy for change in the NHS. The White Paper on quality in this new NHS defines clinical governance in the following terms:

*Clinical governance is a framework through which NHS organisations are accountable for continuously improving the quality of their services and safeguarding high standards of care by creating an environment in which excellence in clinical care will flourish.*

This definition serves to emphasise one of the core difficulties in this field — that of providing an explanation of what the concept entails. The idea for commissioning the papers came directly out of this early challenge. What does clinical governance really mean? What difference will it make to me, to my work and to my 'New NHS'? What do I need to do to rise to its challenge? This book collects together a series of papers which appeared in *Hospital Medicine* over the year or so after that White Paper was published.

A year on, the purpose of the papers is unchanged: to explain clearly and relevantly what clinical governance means to professional practice, whether as an individual practitioner, as a multiprofessional clinical team, or as a whole health care organisation. It also bears emphasis that clinical governance is not new — for as long as clinical practice has existed, the clinical professions have worked to a code governing commonly accepted standards in knowledge, competence and behaviour. What is new is that clinical governance has moved centre stage as an accounting responsibility for any organisation in the NHS.

At the same time, its timing as a policy initiative in our new NHS is vitally important, coming in the aftermath of a series of very prominent cases on professional conduct and performance heard by the General Medical Council, and the introduction of the third major arm of the GMC's work: the new Performance Procedures, introduced from September 1997. Even if this timing is coincidental, there is no doubt that medical practice has never come more acutely under the spotlight of public scrutiny. This public interest has developed a degree of sophistication that the NHS in general and the clinical professions in particular must recognise, understand and respond to. A year on, the public's interest in the way we work and in the quality of our practice is undimmed.

So the present debate on the meaning and management of clinical governance comes at a time when the regulation of the medical profession is under great scrutiny. It is therefore clear that one of the central challenges facing the medical profession today is the need to demonstrate its willingness and capacity to regulate its own practice.

Whether or not the context for clinical governance in the new NHS is focused on perceived deficiency, however, there is no doubt that a culture of governance works best when it is focused on quality improvement and on preventing difficulties arising in the first place. Put another way, instead of having to pull bodies out of a river downstream, we are much better off learning to swim.

An important thread running through these papers is the significance of lifelong learning in supporting a culture of clinical governance. This is not deliverable unless all the stakeholders in clinical practice — whether the individual practitioner, the clinical team, or the whole organisation — are able and willing to make a career-long mutual investment in education, training and professional development.

The most important message, however, is how a culture of clinical governance acts to integrate the elements of an effective health care organisation, how it brings together the evidence that informs clinical practice, the skills that make up clinical competence, and the value set that underpins clinical behaviours, and how it supports individual, team and organisational effectiveness.

When these papers were first published, they presented a series of perspectives of the impact of this new policy initiative on various aspects of clinical life in the NHS. Reflecting the integrating influence of clinical governance, therefore, we felt it important to bring them together as a whole.

*Alastair D Scotland*
*March 2000*
*Director of Medical Education & Research*
*Chelsea & Westminster Healthcare NHS Trust*

# Contributors

Shelley Heard is Dean for Postgraduate Medicine at the Thames Postgraduate Medical and Dental Education, London WC1N 3EJ

Dr Phil Ayres is Medical Director in Medicine, Surgery and Oncology, Leeds Teaching Hospitals NHS Trust, Trust Headquarters, St James's Hospital, Leeds LS9 7TF

Professor Peter Hill is Postgraduate Dean and Director of the Postgraduate Institute for Medicine and Dentistry, University of Newcastle and the NHS Executive Northern and Yorkshire, Newcastle-upon-Tyne NE2 4AB

Dr Peter J Connelly is Consultant Old Age Psychiatrist and Clinical Director of Mental Health, Murray Royal Hospital, Perth PH2 7BH

Professor Ian Haslock is Medical Director in the South Tees Acute Hospitals Trust, South Cleveland Hospital, Middlesbrough TS4 3BW

Dr Stewart Drage is Secretary of the Middlesex Local Medical Committees, Tavistock House, Tavistock Square, London WC1H 9HX

Professor Hilary Thomas is Professor of Oncology at the University of Surrey, Royal Surrey County Hospital, Guildford GU2 5XX

Professor Ian Gilmore is Consultant Physician and Gastroenterologist, Royal Liverpool University Hospitals, and Registrar, Royal College of Physicians, London NW1 4LE

# 1
# Clinical Governance: an opportunity or Pandora's box?

*Shelley Heard*

'Clinical governance? "Ho hum!" you might say – "surely not again"!' It seems that every journal and every conference has this subject as its primary focus. My response is "so they should". The reasons for this come through clearly in the articles in this monograph, which are reproduced from the *Hospital Medicine's* series on clinical governance. A range of perspectives is covered, including the historical and cultural context, the educational perspective, the trust and primary care view and the professional perspective. Different views but, in fact, the same message – clinical governance is the opportunity to get the issue of quality services which address patients needs to the top of the NHS agenda.

## Opportunities and responsibilities

The opportunities afforded by clinical governance are considerable – it potentially enhances, liberates and enables clinicians to lead the healthcare agenda to the benefit of patients. With these opportunities, however, also come responsibilities and the requirement for increased accountability. Professor Hilary Thomas's chapter on revalidation considers more specifically the accountability of doctors within the governance framework and its role to enhancing and securing quality care for patients.

The history of how ideas of quality have developed over the last 20 years is developed by Dr. Phil Ayres. The advance that clinical governance makes over previous quality initiatives is largely one of co-ordinating activities such as clinical risk, clinical audit, evidence based practice, complaints and other quality initiatives. Critically, however, it also acknowledges – possibly for the first time with respect to the quality agenda – the crucial role of leadership and the professional development of staff.

Although the statutory responsibility laid on boards and chief executives for quality is certainly new, most NHS boards and chief executives would have readily acknowledged that the delivery of high quality services was always a key responsibility (Heard, 1999). The multitude of mission statements containing the word 'quality' is a testament to that. The government's new human resources strategy, Working Together: securing a quality workforce,acknowledges that

> *'the link between quality service delivery and quality management of staff is at the heart of all good employment practice'.* (DoH, 1999)

This is perhaps the clearest statement of how the cultural change so clearly the basis of clinical governance is to be achieved.

## Making governance happen

So what is really new about clinical governance? It is its emphasis on professional staff development linked to performance management as a means of developing quality services. Creating a learning environment in the NHS which gives 'permission' for individuals to take seriously their professional development and which makes it necessary for organisations to identify and resource it is an important advance (Heard, 1999). The challenge will be whether the government is serious about resources being used in this way since either new, additional resources will have to be identified or current resources will need to be diverted from direct patient care in order to support staff development. However it is to be done, the patient should ultimately benefit since as Professor Peter Hill points out

> *'clinical governance offers a real chance to enhance the quality of patient care. It provides a coherent framework within which education and training can be directed towards this particular goal.' (Hill, 1999)*

Will the government and patient groups be persuaded that this is really the case? There will need to be a debate over whether it is the quantum or the quality of healthcare that matters. Inevitably a balance will need to be struck which will enable healthcare staff to have sufficient time and resource to ensure that the necessary opportunities are available for them to pursue the professional development they require to support modern, evidence informed patient care. Is this a good enough reason to extend waiting lists and waiting times? Will the public buy into their responsibilities and give support to this initiative? When a patient comes into a general practitioner's surgery with all of the latest information from the net – having spent hours 'surfing' in order to become expert on their own medical condition – there is an expectation that the doctor will have done the same. In a perfect world this would certainly be the case. But in a world of six and a half minute consultations and high patient/carer expectations there will be costs which need to become acceptable to patients and to the NHS if the governance agenda is to be implemented. It may be early days for patient participation in such questions (Dewar, 1999) but frameworks to involve them will need to be developed. Primary care has a unique opportunity to imbed both the principles and practice of clinical governance into the emerging organisations of primary care – initially primary care groups (PCGs) and then primary care trusts (PCTs). Dr. Stuart Drage explores clinical governance with the context of primary care the potential opportunities it offers to improve care for patients.

## Approaches to governance

Strategies to implement clinical governance are being developed regionally and within healthcare organisations. The Department of Health's most recent guidance, Clinical Governance: quality in the New NHS, makes clear that

> *'above all clinical governance is about changing organisational culture in a systematic and demonstrable way, moving away from a culture of "blame" to one of learning so that quality infuses all aspects of the organisation's work"* (DoH, 1999).

This is indeed a profound statement that is explored in the context of mental health practice in Dr. Peter Connelly's chapter. The use of a *'local team implementation plan'* acknowledges the place of the healthcare team in managing patient issues and the need for team members to respect each other and their role in the team in order to achieve maximum benefit for the patient. Professor Ian Haslock, medical director at South Tees, describes the use of the European Quality Foundation model that was introduced into the trust in order to provide a framework for quality development. With the strong and personal commitment of the Chief Executive, South Tees has positioned itself to address the requirements of clinical governance. Embedding a belief in the essential *'rightness'* of governance into organisations will require however, the commitment of everyone since as Haslock points out, *'we are all in this together'*.

## Opportunity or Pandora's box?

Clinical governance potentially presents an opportunity that could liberate and enable the NHS to become the best that it can be. It is a fitting gift to the NHS in its fiftieth year, since it restates and invigorates the values of its foundation. But it could turn out to be a Pandora's box, creating more problems than solutions, more trouble for staff and patients than support and more tension in the delivery of healthcare than resolution of difficult issues. Which way it will go will depend on the success of the partnerships that can be created. Partnerships not only of healthcare and other professionals, but partnerships between politics and health and critically, between the people and health. Professor Ian Gilmore explores some of these partnerships in the final chapter of this monograph.

Health is a political issue. The opportunity offered by clinical governance is that it opens the debate on quality – what it is and critically, how it is to be achieved. If the public want a health service which is about access and equity, but which is also about excellence then it – and its political representatives – must be prepared to consider what this really means. It may mean hospitals which are larger groups of clinical teams, resulting in the closure of smaller, local services; it may mean longer waits for some clinical procedures or the cessation of some procedures all together if the evidence for undertaking them is insufficient; it will certainly require greater investment and care for the healthcare professionals who deliver the service and who are committed to ensuring that it continues to develop to the benefit of patient care.

## Key Points

- Clinical governance brings with it both opportunities and responsibilities.

- Focussing and co-ordinating quality initiatives are major components of developing clinical governance.

- The emphasis on staff development and learning as a means of developing quality services is the really new aspect of clinical governance.

- The tension between the quantum of healthcare delivered and its quality requires public debate and resolution

- Debate over how quality through governance is to be achieved must include its political dimension.

- Partnerships between health, politics and the public will be required to necessary if clinical governance is to be implemented.

## References

Department of Health (1999) *Working Together – securing a quality workforce for the NHS. HSC 1999/079.* Department of Health,Leeds

Dewar S (1999) *Clinical governance under construction.* The King's Fund, London

Department of Health (1999) *Clinical governance: quality in the new NHS. HSC 1999/065.* Department of Health, Leeds

Heard S (1997) Quality healthcare: the hospital chief executive's role. *Quality in Health Care* **8**:99–101

Heard S (1998) Educating towards clinical governance. *Hospital Medicine* **59**:728–9

Hill P (1999) Clinical governance: an educational perspective. *Hospital Medicine* **60**:596–8

# 2
# Clinical governance: setting the scene

*Phil Ayres*

Clinical governance first appeared as part of official UK Government policy on the publication of the White Paper *The New NHS: Modern, Dependable* in December 1997 (NHS Executive, 1997). Further guidance was issued in the publication of *A First Class Service* (NHS Executive, 1998) in July 1998 and, more recently, direct guidance on clinical governance from the NHS Executive was published (NHS Executive, 1999). There is still, however, uncertainty about what clinical governance means and how it should be implemented.

This chapter describes the origins of clinical governance by referring to previous quality initiatives in the NHS. It demonstrates how these have been joined together in a single focus for quality improvement under the new banner of clinical governance. The chapter concludes with the notion that the clinical governance bandwagon should be carrying as many managers as clinicians.

## How do we know if a service is any good?

Clinical services may be seen by health professionals as a product of daily activity. To patients they are a series of meetings and acquaintances, interventions and outcomes that may lead to a 'good' or 'bad' result. A crude example of a service is shown in *Figure 1.1*

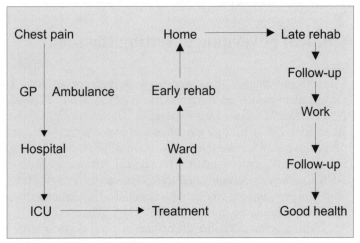

**Figure 1.1: Example of a clinical service**

In this example a patient experiences chest pain and hopefully ends up in good health. The journey of the patient runs through primary care, ambulance services, acute and rehabilitation departments of a hospital, outpatient follow-up, return to work and eventually discharge from the health services' attention.

Deciding whether or not the service which the patient experiences is any good has become a complex task. In the past 20 years we have attempted to address issues of quality through a number of different initiatives. These are shown in *Figure 1.2*.

| | |
|---|---|
| Resource Management | Mid 1980s |
| Quality | 1990 |
| Clinical Audit (originally medical | 1991 |
| Patients' Charter | 1993 |
| Clinical Guidelines | 1993 onwards |
| Clinical Effectiveness | 1995 |
| Clinical Governance | 1997 |

*Figure 1.2: History of clinical governance*

Each of these initiatives has attempted to focus on different aspects of the patient journey. Unfortunately they are now seen with some scepticism as failures. But the need for quality and control in these areas remains, and it is for this reason that they have all effectively been amalgamated in the guise of clinical governance. Each of the initiatives will be discussed briefly in turn.

## Resource management

The Resource Management Initiative (RMI) was a popular approach with NHS managers in the mid–late 1980s. It legitimized the role of managers in asking questions about how effectively resources (financial, facilities, personnel) were being used. Demonstration sites were established in different parts of the UK and groups where there was access to high quality information. This information was used to liaise directly with clinicians on how to change resource use. Some useful work was undertaken but wholesale change in the way the professions and managers approached the whole agenda of health-care provision did not materialize. With the NHS reforms of 1990, the quality agenda and medical audit were about to take over.

## Quality

Quality was made everyone's business with the 1990 reforms. Directors of quality, or an explicit role for quality resting with the Chief Nurse, became commonplace in NHS trusts and directly managed units (DMUs). No overall approach to the management of quality was openly commended to the NHS by the NHS Management Executive. In many trusts and DMUs, useful work in partnership with professionals was undertaken by management groups, in the name of quality. However, fully integrated approaches to understanding and managing the quality agenda were not commonplace and clinicians (particularly medical) were about to have the quality agenda refocused in terms of medical audit.

## Medical audit

Medical audit was initially designed as a peer review process which would be mandatory for doctors. Time was allocated for the pursuit of medical audit projects. Large amounts of cash were made available to hospitals to develop audit departments. Newly appointed audit facilitators helped to oil the wheels. Over time, medical audit changed to clinical audit and the other professions were brought in, not only to have access to the funds, but also to participate actively with doctors in taking decisions about quality.

But there was little enthusiasm for change and many have reported on the inability of the clinical audit process alone to deliver significant improvements in health services (NHS Confederation, 1997). However, although the demise of clinical audit has long been forecast, health professionals still regard it as a useful tool in the management of quality. Subsequent initiatives (see below) have reinforced the need for a high quality clinical audit programme and this is also evident in current clinical governance policy.

## Patients' Charter

A further dimension to the quality agenda was introduced in terms of statutory duties for trusts for certain aspects of care delivery (eg. waiting lists). Targets were set and chief executive performance was managed taking into account how far Patients' Charter targets had been met. Also the subject of much criticism, the Patients' Charter movement was represented by a series of highly focused activities which culminated in 'returns' which were scrutinised by managers and administrators elsewhere. The emphasis on patient choice and patient-focused decision taking was lost.

## Clinical guidelines

The evidence-based medicine movement (Sackett and Haynes, 1995) and a desire (largely in America) to see that health resources were spent wisely, resulted in a massive effort to generate and implement clinical guidelines in the early and mid 1990s. The National Institute for Health in the USA set up bodies specifically to develop guidelines by which the practice of clinicians could be codified and judged.

The movement quickly spread to the rest of the world and the guidelines movement in the UK, coupled with other international initiatives such as the Cochrane Collaboration, provided an evidence base for some aspects of clinical practice.

Researchers began to conduct studies which looked at how to successfully implement clinical guidelines and much of this evidence has recently been summarized (NHS Centre for Reviews and Dissemination, 1999). We now know what to do to change professional practice when there is clear evidence that we should do so.

## Clinical effectiveness

Clinical effectiveness was widely seen as the successor to clinical audit. It involved a more comprehensive approach (Ayres *et al*, 1996) which encompassed many other determinants of outcome. The building blocks of clinical effectiveness are shown in *Table 1.1*.

In reality a much narrower definition was implied by much of the activity underpinning clinical effectiveness programmes. These were:

- evidence-based practice activities (Sackett and Haynes, 1995)
- the development of (but often failure to imclinical guidelines
- more clinical audit.

| Table 1.1: Clinical effectiveness |
|---|
| Accessing the evidence: proper use of libraries |
| Applying the principles of evidence-based health care to clinical practice |
| Using information technology to improve clinical decision |
| Developing clinical audit |
| Clinical guidelines — appropriate use |
| Clinical risk management |
| Effective professional education |
| Research and development |
| Promoting dialogue between primary and secondary care and public health |
| Involving patients |
| Effective senior management |

## Putting it all together

A summary of characteristics of all the initiatives described so far is shown in *Table 1.2*. By putting all of these together, we demonstrate how, individually, they contributed to a better understanding of the overall patient care process (*Figure 1.3*).

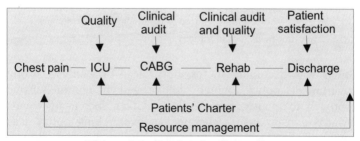

***Figure 1.3: Putting it all together***

| Table 1.2: Summary of initiatives looking at quality | |
|---|---|
| RMI | To develop, in conjuntion with clinical staff, local management processes for planning and controlling the use of resources |
| Quality | 'Directorys of Quality' created<br>'Total quality management' of importance<br>Patient satisfaction given high priority |
| Clinical audit | The audit cycle of reviewing practice<br>Setting standards<br>Making changes<br>Reviewing practice brought into common use |
| Patient's Charter | Rigidly defined criteria (eg. Number of patients waiting 18 months<br>League tables<br>CEO performance managed by this<br>Charter Units developed |
| Clinical guidelines | Formal standard setting<br>Uses rigorous processes<br>Evidence based methods<br>Seen as controlling local clinical activity<br>Local ownership of process required<br>Known to be effective at improving outcomes<br>Development and implementation |
| Clinical effectiveness | Seen as successor to clinical audit<br>An organization goal in itself<br>Barriers to successful implementation not clearly understood<br>Sometimes criticized as manipulating professionals |
| RMI = resource management initiative | |

But it was becoming increasingly clear that only a strong government policy, which emphasized a comprehensive approach to quality, was required. Given increasing trends towards consumerism generally, an overarching policy was bound to emerge. It is not surprising that when clinical governance appeared in NHS policy documents, its first point was to suggest the coordination of quality initiatives as well as other tasks (*Table 1.3*).

| Table 1.3: Clinical governance |
|---|
| Coordinate quality drives |
| Develop leaders of clinical services |
| Evidence-based practice |
| Dissemination of good practice and innovation |
| Clinical risk management |
| Clinical performance management |
| Professional development programmes |
| Information systems needed to support clinical governance |

## The emergence of clinical governance

The term clinical governance was coined in the White Paper published by the Labour government in December 1997. Professor Liam Donaldson, now the Chief Medical Officer, is largely credited as the originator of the term and the overall shape of the policy.

If to coordinate quality initiatives is one task of clinical governance, then the other tasks should fall into place (*Table 1.3*). The resulting programme of work would be expected to be driven by management. Indeed, the overall responsibility for clinical governance rests with trust chief executives: increasing the notion that this is a management agenda (even though this will ultimately mean managing clinical staff). But the emergence of the policy has coincided with a series of very public and acrimonious engagements between the medical profession, the General Medical Council, the media and some patients or their carers. As a result, a lot of emphasis has been placed on the medical profession's role in the delivery of clinical governance. The role of management remains unclear, but implications for the 'policing' of the medical and other professions have been widely reported in the professional and lay press. Suspicion about the NHS management's motives for the clinical governance agenda is growing.

## Supporting the initiative

Lack of clarity about the role of management has therefore become a two-edged outcome. On the one hand, few components of government policy have been as well-publicized, and few clinicians have escaped at least hearing about clinical governance. On the other hand, the steps which management must take to support the development of clinical governance are being developed in an ad hoc fashion, not on a national basis.

Managerialism is, however, taking an ever-higher profile in the NHS, and sooner or later we will see the NHS Executive introduce guidance on management effectiveness. Models abound, but a favourite is thought to be that of the European Foundation for Quality Management: the Business Excellence Model (*Figure 1.4*).

This model was developed by a collaboration of industry-based concerns, which realized that getting quality right not only provides the competitive edge, but is actually the key to survival.

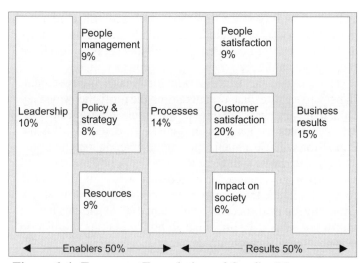

***Figure 1.4: European Foundation of Quality Management:
Business Excellence Model***

The challenge for NHS management becomes twofold:

- to set clear goals and national standards for management effectiveness
- to engage clinical staff using methods of support, rather than sanction, to achieve the aims of the clinical governance agenda.

## Monitoring progress

Nationally, two new institutions are being created to support clinical governance. The first, the National Institute for Clinical

Excellence, will produce rigorous guidance for clinicians, using evidence-based methods. It is likely that these reviews and guidelines will be collated from existing sources, so a huge bureaucracy is unlikely.

The second, the Commission for Health Improvement, will help to ensure that organizations perform the way they should. This massive agenda will inevitably focus on how far chief executives have a grip on quality. To determine this the Commission will use annual reports, and other documentation.

In future, trusts will have to report in public on how well their clinical governance arrangements are working. These reports will include the arrangements for managing clinical risk and monitoring professional performance. That patients have a 'right to know' is ever prevalent in policy making: a position that is proving difficult to argue against.

## Conclusion

We have seen clinical governance develop from the first efforts of the NHS to create policy which controls resource use and satisfies the public's demand for ever greater access to, and quality of, health care. Historical initiatives have met with limited success, but each of these has been brought together in the guise of clinical governance to form a global approach to quality management which clinicians and managers are not permitted to opt out of.

The agenda is complex, requiring action at the team, local, district, regional, and national levels. The work to be done is not yet as clear as it needs to be, but the change is coming. Effective action by managers to support clinicians is vital.

The inevitable conclusion is that the key to success is organisational focus. Together, managers and professionals need to focus on the patient's perspective in everything that they do. Achieving that is another story all together.

## Key Points

- Clinical governance has grown from a number of NHS policy initiatives over the last 10 years

- Clinical governance is about quality

- Effective mamnagement involvement is essential, especially in a supporting role

- Clinical governance is not an option: eventually we will all be 'measured' under its auspices

- Focusing clinical terms on the patient's perspective will deliver much of what is intended

## References

Ayres PJ, Wright J, Donaldson LJ (1996) Achieving clinical effectiveness: the new world of clinical governance. *Clinician in Management* **7**: 106–11

NHS Centre for Reviews and Dissemination (1999) Getting evidence into practice. *Effective Health Care* **5**(1)

NHS Confederation (1997) *Acting on the Evidence: Progress in the NHS.* NHS Confederation, Birmingham

NHS Executive (1997) *The New NHS: Modern,Dependable.* HMSO, London

NHS Executive (1998) *A First Class Service.* HMSO, London

NHS Executive (1999) *Clinical Governance: Quality in the New NHS.* HSC 1999/065. HMSO, London

Sackett DL, Haynes RB (1995) On the need for evidence-based medicine. *Evidence-Based Medicine* **1**: 5–6

# 3
# Clinical governance: an educational perspective

*Peter Hill*

Clinical governance is a central plank of government policy to put quality at the heart of the NHS (Department of Health, 1997). This chapter looks at what this means for the health service, and highlights some of the educational implications.

## The current context

Great forces for change are fundamentally affecting the health service and the way we work within it. These include the rapid expansion of knowledge and possible skills, the revolution in technology which continually pushes out boundaries, and the increasing involvement in health care of a wider range of health professionals, accompanied by increasing complexity. Patients are demanding a much greater role. Doctors also desire a life outside of medicine.

## The concept

Clinical governance is a breathtaking idea, whose simplicity belies its complexity; many people outside the NHS are surprised at the lack of responsibility for its quality within the NHS at present.

The term is derived from the commercial world following a number of high profile institutional failures with significant losses of investor funds, and stems from the Cadbury report

(Cadbury, 1992) now widely adopted in the public sector. In relation to hospitals the term is much older, going back to 1660 (Coke, 1992). In a modern context it can be viewed at three levels: strategic, systems and operational.

## The strategic imperative

The consistent provision of high quality clinical care will only happen if there are effective partnerships between health professionals and managers within NHS organizations. For these to develop, major cultural changes need to occur. Doctors need to have respect for and trust other professionals and health service managers. Much will depend on the approach and style adopted by the fledgling clinical governance structures being established. If doctors (and other health professional staff) are not adequately trained or continually updated then patients, and the NHS trust responsible for their care, are at risk. These attitudes need fostering, including through multidisciplinary, multiprofessional training. Those involved in the management and delivery of postgraduate training therefore need including in relevant partnerships within the wider NHS and at strategic levels.

## The systems dimension

Clinical governance means integrating a number of existing systems, including clinical audit, the handling of complaints and clinical risk management, well described by the British Association of Medical Managers (1998). New systems also need to be developed and put in place. Lines of accountability need to be clearly defined. Good practice and evidence-based innovations will be systematically disseminated and implemented.

## At the sharp end: the operational dimension

To embed clinical governance in routine medical practice, doctors need appropriate attitudes, knowledge and skills. At present much time and effort is expended in inculcating trainees with (perfectly appropriate) specialist elements relevant to their chosen specialty and future clinical practice. To enable them to meet their responsibilities for clinical governance they also need to work in teams, be constantly constructively self critical (and hence play a full and proper part in clinical audit), be committed to continuing professional development (CPD), know how to avail themselves of and apply relevant best evidence, and meet the responsibilities set out in Good Medical Practice (General Medical Council (GMC), 1998a).

## Patients and doctors in the future

To consider what sort of doctor the NHS should develop for the next millennium we must look at the patient of the future since we are in the business of meeting their health needs.

Patients will be knowledgeable because they are increasingly better educated and have more access to the growing tide of information available through the media, the Internet and other sources. As a consequence they will have high expectations, and want much more of a partnership with doctors and other health professionals involved in their care. *'Do as I tell you'* and *'Trust me, I'm a doctor'* approaches will no longer endure. Patients are already more willing to complain.

Just as the information available to patients grows, so the knowledge and potential skills for doctors to acquire is expanding. Doctors of the future will be lifelong learners and evidence-based practitioners. Every doctor will need to be clinically competent and perform consistently well. While practising ethically and protecting patients from harm, future practitioners will need to contribute to care as effective team players. They will need to be committed to teaching and training, clinical audit and research, and maintain CPD with regular revalidation.

CPD has been defined as:

> *'a process of lifelong learning for all individuals and teams which meets the needs of patients and delivers the health outcomes and healthcare priorities of the NHS and which enables professionals to expand and fulfil their potential.'* (Department of Health, 1998)

## The lifelong learner: a professional continuum

Lifelong learning should involve a systematic approach whereby doctors and other health professionals are helped to identify development needs that would enable them to do their jobs better (ie. raise its quality) and move them towards career goals they may have (*Figure 2.1*). This is a laudable aim to be welcomed in the recently published NHS human resource strategy (NHS Executive, 1998). Postgraduate medical organizations are well placed to play a crucial part.

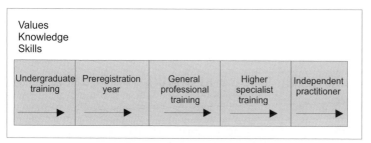

Values
Knowledge
Skills

| Undergraduate training | Preregistration year | General professional training | Higher specialist training | Independent practitioner |

***Figure 2.1: The life long learner —
a professional continuum***

Personal development plans (PDPs) should be seen as a helpful tool in this postgraduate education process. Elements should identify the service goals to be addressed (for example, through the acquisition or development of clinical or other skills) and career aspirations, how needs could be met, the timescale for achievement, and how success will be judged. The issue of resources cannot be ignored.

The principles behind, and key components of, PDPs should be common to all NHS staff. It is their content, arrived at by joint discussions and negotiation, that will differ. Initially plans are likely to focus on what could or should be achieved perhaps within the next 3 years.

This process would be a big step in helping to foster links between clinical governance, lifelong learning and evidence-based practice, since the latter must be at the heart of many professional development initiatives.

Currently my perception is of much time and resource wasted on courses of doubtful provenance and value, with no predetermined objectives or follow-up regarding improvements in skills or competencies, let alone service or health gain.

As a postgraduate dean providing funding I feel I am often supporting one of the provincial railway companies, and hotels and other organizations in the south-east of England.

## Linking education and training, and quality of care

High quality care depends on sound education and training (GMC, 1998b). All experienced doctors have a responsibility for the personal and professional development of trainees with whom they work, as role models, teachers and supervisors. The Calman reforms to specialist training, in my view, offer the best opportunity to meet trainees' educational needs. The structures and processes are largely in place; the challenge is to equip those managing and delivering education and training to fulfil this promise. Trainees should expect:

- educational supervision
- clinical supervision
- personal training objectives
- regular review of their learning needs and plans
- feedback on performance
- an induction programme at every new location
- systematic clinical training, with generic and specialist components
- access to evidence
- access to advice and support.

Trainees must have educational and clinical supervision appropriate to their experience and which helps their personal and professional development. Their training, wherever and whenever possible, should be tailored to individual needs. They need positive and constructive negative feedback on their performance. A balance must be struck between the specialty component of training and the broader range of skills and experience needed to equip them to be effective consultants. All health professionals need access to the evidence they need to care for patients properly day and night. Trainees also need ready access to a range of advice and support.

Consultant trainers need to support and help trainees meet these aspirations. We have some way to go to reach the full application of equal opportunities principles. To learn and maximize the opportunities available, expectations must be made explicit at every stage. Service interactions are arguably the best for learning and should be exploited as fully as possible.

However, trainees have responsibilities too. They must comply with Good Medical Practice (GMC, 1998a), they also have to work and they must take responsibility for their own CPD. Gatrell and White (1999) have gone a long way to providing a comprehensive self driven approach.

## Professional self-regulation at a local level

Professional self-regulation at a local level will be an essential part of arrangements for clinical governance (Scally and Donaldson, 1998). This key element will have national approaches and statutory bodies acting in support. Local measures must be in place when it is identified that trainee doctors or established practitioners need to improve performance. Team work will be essential, as will the cooperation of individuals identified and their colleagues.

## The patient perspective

Increasing the input of patients and the public to all aspects of the service is another central government aim. This notion needs to permeate every aspect of the NHS, from the consultation (at its heart, surely the central task of medicine) outwards. Achieving this will not be easy, but the first important step is to make the commitment to do so. To engage the public more closely in clinical governance, one approach for those of us involved in (postgraduate medical) education would be to elicit patient views on how they perceive their care by doctors in training.

## So what needs to happen?

While the quest for quality stimulated by clinical governance is laudable, there are considerable resource implications that need recognizing at a national level by the government.

For trusts this is another important strand in an already crowded agenda, but which will be underpinned by a statutory responsibility. It needs constructive action and interaction between health professionals and managers internally and, in the field of education and training, externally with postgraduate medical organizations and other education providers.

All doctors need to be aware of their responsibilities for the care of patients and education and training as part of CPD. Where needs are identified doctors must avail themselves of opportunities to meet those needs. The role of postgraduate medical education organizations, and part of my responsibility, is to ensure such opportunities are available.

## Conclusions

Clinical governance offers a real chance to enhance the quality of patient care. It provides a coherent framework within which education and training can be directed towards this goal.

### Key points

- Clinical governance is a new approach to quality with profound implications

- Patients of the future will expect and demand high quality care

- High quality education and training underpins high quality care

- Doctors must become lifelong learners and evidence-based practitioners

- Trainers and trainees have expectations and responsibilities

- Action needs to be taken at national, local and individual levels

## References

British Association of Medical Managers (1998) *Clinical Governance in the new NHS.* BAMM, Cheadle

Cadbury, Sir A (1992) *Report of the Committee on the Financial Aspects of Corporate Governance.* Gee, London

Coke R (1992) Of the Foundation, Erection and Governance of Hospitals. In: *The Shorter Oxford English Dictionary.* Oxford University Press, Oxford

Department of Health (1997) *The New NHS: modern-dependable.* HMSO, London

Department of Health (1998) *A First Class Service: quality in the new NHS.* HMSO, London

Gatrell J, White T (1999) *The Specialist Registrar Handbook*. Radcliffe
    Medical Press, Oxford

General Medical Council (1998a) *Good Medical Practice. GMC*, London

General Medical Council (1998b) *The Early Years*. GMC, London

NHS Executive (1998) *Working together - securing a quality workforce for
    the NHS*. HSC 1998/162. Department of Health, London

Scally G, Donaldson LJ (1998) Clinical governance and the drive for
    quality improvement in the new NHS in England. *Br Med J*
    **317**:61–5

# 4
# What will we do without to get what we really want?

*Peter J Connelly*

In 1998, Sam Galbraith, Minister of Health for Scotland, said: *'The best definition that I have seen of clinical governance is simply that it means "corporate accountability for clinical performance".'* The context of this interpretation of clinical governance should not be overlooked. Comparisons can be made with corporate governance and its financial focus. It is important that clinical governance is not simply the introduction of control mechanisms and quality assurance, but that a 'hearts and minds' change in the culture of delivering health services accompanies this accountability (British Association of Medical Managers, 1998).

## A 'hearts and minds' change

> That patient should never have absconded. Carry out an investigation of how it could possibly happen. Someone must be to blame — we are always putting extra resources into that ward. Discipline is required here.

This scenario is likely to be all too familiar to a number of readers, but is it really clinical governance in action?

Why were extra resources required in the ward? Was this a permanent increase in staffing, multiple temporary moves, or an indication that something serious was wrong in the ward? If there are difficult patients, is there a pool of sufficiently trained nurses to carry out functions which are clearly over and above

*33*

the workload involved in the day-to-day management of patients?

In the setting of low morale and under-staffing it is difficult to maintain a quality service. Have adequate steps been taken to identify the root of this perception and to resolve the problems? Is team building working optimally? The ward environment may not be conducive to the therapeutic management of patients. Has there been sufficient investment in the fabric of the ward to raise its therapeutic potential?

## Clinical governance: a new framework

An initial response to the challenges of clinical governance has often revolved around more accurate counting of data and the setting up of a committee to oversee the process primarily geared towards the need to 'target bad apples', including adequate sanctions for dealing with practitioners who are under-performing and emphasizing the rather reactive nature of risk management. In fact, this is an extreme over- simplification of the change in culture required to ensure successful governance.

In reality, most clinicians (of all disciplines) already deliver a high quality service under considerable pressure. An atmosphere of encouragement rather than criticism should drive clinical governance if people are to admit to poor quality and to learn from errors. Fundamental to successful implementation of clinical governance is that the culture of examining practice in the NHS changes with a change in ethos to concentrate on the questions 'Are we doing the right thing?', 'If so, are we doing it right?', and 'What will we do without to get what we really want?'. The desired outcomes are increased involvement, increased ownership, increased morale and increased expertise among NHS staff.

## Clinical risk assessment and management

Fundamental to governance is the identification and reduction of clinical risk. Risk cannot be eliminated and indeed is inherent in psychiatry, where the patient's behaviour is modified by the illness itself, and where poor peer support has contributed to adverse learning before coming into contact with the mental health services. Risk is dynamic and prone to change; with some patients this can be rapid. Intervention can increase as well as decrease risk. Accurate assessment of risk is crucially dependent upon the interaction between the clinician and the patient. Even after rigorous assessment outcomes can be unpredictable. Some people are liable to abscond, no matter what relationship they have with staff.

Assessment of risk will vary between specialities but in mental health, current mental state and social circumstances will be greater determinants of risk than previous history, even though the latter may include violence or suicidal behaviour.

In formulating the risk, questions should address the seriousness, the immediacy and the specific nature of the risk before formulating a management plan. Such management will encompass a range of professionals and information needs to be passed clearly between individuals.

Equity of assessment and response is required. Staff must not simply prioritize potential risks of patient violence or absconding in young people but must ensure that clinical risks are not underestimated in older people.

Managing risk is not a simple matter. A law of diminishing returns applies. Hypothetically, in a ward with 20 staff, six incidents of absconding might be expected per year; with 40 staff two incidents might be expected, but even with 80 staff an incident might occur. A balance is required but both management and staff must accept that some incidents will occur and that additional staff will not always be a solution. How should managers respond, however, if staff in the ward at the outset of this article demonstrate that incidents are 90% lower with six on a shift than with five?

To ensure that clinical risk management works well, ensure that people are working within their level of competence. Staff are unlikely to be complacent about absconding, but a culture of 'no blame' requires development where practical, with systems in place to deal with poor practice. This involves openness, monitoring, appraisal and re-training where required. Standards, guidelines and protocols require agreement and review with the concept of the Local Team Implementation Plan (LIP) being developed to ensure an integration of training, easier objective setting and appraisal.

## Multidisciplinary clinical risk assessment

Consider the following conversation between a physiotherapist, nurse and occupational therapist in a dementia ward.

> 'There's no point in having that patient sitting in that chair — his posture is inappropriate and his mobility will deteriorate. He will be in hospital longer than necessary' says the physiotherapist.

'But his agitation is more severe if he is not in that chair and he is at risk of more falls and will be in hospital longer than necessary' says the nurse, 'Perhaps medication would help.'

'There's no point in giving him more medication', says the occupational therapist, 'I won't be able to work with him and he will be in hospital longer than necessary'.

How would such an apparent 'no-win' situation be resolved to the benefit of the patient? Within a LIP focused on improving rehabilitation of agitated patients at risk of falling, the mixture of mobilization, exercise and therapeutic input can be adjusted to allow the patient to gain the benefits of relaxing in a suitable chair without periods of prolonged inactivity or increase in medication.

## Improving practice

### Clinical guidelines

There are many definitions of guidelines, of which the Evidence-based Medicine Working Group (Hayward *et al*, 1995) is probably the most pragmatic. The problems for which guidelines are most needed are complex trade-offs between competing benefits, harm and costs, usually under conditions of uncertainty. While there has been resistance to the introduction of guidelines, which are perceived by some as inhibiting clinical practice, most conditions in psychiatry fulfil the criteria for which guidelines are most needed.

Guidelines provide a focus for two mechanisms closely associated with clinical governance: clinical audit and integrated care pathways (ICPs).

## Clinical audit

Suspicions about the motivation behind developing guidelines and the motivation of commissioners in seeking audit has led to an inconsistent approach to the topic throughout the country, which must change.

CRAG, in its paper The Interface between Audit and Management (Clinical Resource and Audit Group, 1993), highlights some very useful conditions for audit. Ideally, audit should involve issues which are common problems, a significant or serious condition, relevant to the team's or individual's practice or need for development. Potential directions for change should be identified which are likely to bring benefits to patients or greater effectiveness in the delivery of care. There should be a realistic potential for improvement in the service and the end result should justify the time and effort in the process.

## Integrated care pathways

Guidelines and audit based around them can combine to ensure standards are met and allow the development of appropriate protocols.

ICPs require the development of common practices which should enhance the communication between members of an effective clinical team. They can be an effective alternative to multiple unidisciplinary care plans and allow common milestones in the treatment of patients to be identified thus allowing exceptions to be recorded making audit, critical incident review and targeted training easier to conduct.

Clear lines of accountability are required which may well be a potent issue in a multidisciplinary, multi-agency approach such as that commonly seen in psychiatry. Each member of the team must be aware of the need for exception reporting, and be committed to using that information to drive clinical audit and to make clinical risk management more effective.

## Critical incident analysis

Even the most successful guidelines, protocols, ICPs, audit and risk management procedures will be unable to prevent all incidents occurring. An effective clinical team will be aware of the need to investigate critical incidents:

- speedily — memory is fresh
- sensitively — people are feeling vulnerable
- scrupulously — to identify issues which may affect future patient care
- supportively — ensuring a culture of openness and lack of apportioning blame is at the heart of team-working.

## Effective clinical team

Crucial to clinical governance is the ability to develop strong and effective clinical teams with clear leadership. The rewards are better multidisciplinary integration, better joint planning and better integration with other agencies. Effective teams cannot function without committed, supportive management, without time to be properly professional with patients and without resources to make self regulation work well.

## Managing poor performance

Inevitably some critical incidents will be a result of poor performance, although this will not be the only manifestation of a poorly performing individual or team. A clear structure must be in place to identify and manage performance including transparent disciplinary measures if required. However, an effective clinical team will benefit from the use of internal and external appraisal of performance.

# Appraisal

A system of appraisal is required to identify opportunities for improving performance, marrying personal development, service development and overall management of service resources. This combination of approach ensures that service innovations become common practice and that training is tailored to improving performance. As an example, widening the consultant job plan to include issues which affect performance, including non-clinical aspects of a consultant's job, is an ideal vehicle on which to base a system of appraisal, in which use of service resources, development of staff, targeted continuing professional development and monitoring of involvement outwith normal clinical remit can be discussed openly (BMA Central Consultants and Specialists Committee, 1998).

An agreed balance between existing tasks and the incorporation of new tasks is required reflecting the needs of the trust and the development of individual consultants. Prioritization requires a key question — 'What must we do without to get what we really want?'

## Barriers to governance

External barriers to successful governance exist. These include a poor fabric of building in which to deliver inpatient services, too few alternatives to admission, too few treatment options and too little integration of multidisciplinary follow-up.

Conditions which can lead to errors happening include high workload, too much complacency or exhaustion, inadequate knowledge, ability or experience to manage conditions, poor design, inadequate supervision or instruction, a stressful environment and too much or too little change!

These factors affect commissioners who again must ask 'What will we do without to get what we really want?'

## Implementation plans

The development of Service Implementation Plans and LIPs will enhance the implementation of governance in areas in which multidisciplinary and multiagency work is common, such as mental health, with agreed training and targeted areas for improvement of care, allowing exploration of relationships within departments as well.

## Successful governance

In summary, to change from existing practices to a new form of successful clinical governance in mental health services, the development of LIPs, focusing on the questions 'Are we doing the right thing?', 'If so, are we doing it right?', and 'What will we do without to get what we really want?' provide a sound basis for improvement.

The keys to success are a willingness to pursue a hearts and minds change, a mature approach to clinical risk assessment and management, developing appropriate clinical guidelines, audit and ICPs without stifling innovation, learning from critical incident analysis, developing team-focused objectives and appraisal, managing poor performance and removing barriers to governance; something which involves not only service providers but commissioners too.

### Key points

- Good clinical governance requires an atmospher of encouragement rather than criticism if people are to admit to poor quality and learn from errors.

- Key questions are 'Are we doing the right thing?', 'If so, are we doing it right?' and 'What will we do without to get what we really what?'

- Fundamental to clinical governance is the multidisciplinary identification and reduction of clinical risk.

- Risk is dynamic and prone to change.

- Developing a Local Team Implementation Plan ensures integration of training, easier objective setting and appraisal.

- Guidelines, care pathways and audit form a natural progression which underpins clinical governance.

- Strong and effective clinical teams with clear evidence of leadership are crucial to the whole ethos of clinical governance.

- A clear structure must be in place to identify and manage performance including transparent disciplinary measures if these are required.

- External barriers to governance must be dealt with to improve implementation.

- Governance involves not only service providers but commissioners too.

# References

BMA Central Consultants and Specialists Committee (CCSC) (1998) *Appraisal for Senior Hospital Doctors.* British Medical Association, London

British Association of Medical Managers (1998) *Clinical Governance — A Document for Consultation.* British Association of Medical Managers, Cheadle, Cheshire

Clinical Resource and Audit Group (1993) *The Interface between Clinical Audit and Management.* Clinical Resource and Audit Group, Scottish Office, Edinburgh

Galbraith S (1998) *NHS MEL (1998) 75.* Scottish Office Department of Health, Edinburgh

Hayward RS, Wilson MC, Tunis SR, Bass EB, Guyatt G (1995) Users guide to medical literature VIII. How to use clinical practice guidelines A. Are the recommendations valid? *JAMA* **274**:570–4

# 5
# Introducing clinical governance in an acute trust

*Ian Haslock*

Clinical governance can be defined as a framework through which NHS organizations are accountable for continuously improving the quality of their services and safeguarding high standards of care, by creating an environment in which excellence in clinical care will flourish (Department of Health, 1998). This definition of clinical governance encompasses two distinct elements — the mechanistic element of ensuring systems are in place, and the more philosophical element of producing a culture in which clinical quality can flourish.

This chapter describes the approach to these challenges used by a large acute trust which provides acute services to a population of over 300000, tertiary services to a population of about 1 million and employs more than 4600 staff, of whom 170 are consultants. Our aim was to take a snapshot of the trust as it is at present, and to use the results to ask two questions: do we have the right culture, and do we have the right structures?

## Do we have the right culture?

South Tees Acute Hospitals Trust was a second-wave trust which has prided itself in its commitment to quality. What is the evidence for this? Four elements stand out: the Trust's mission statement, its definition of its core values, the use of the European Quality Foundation model for developing excellence and the commitment of key staff to quality improvement.

## The Trust's mission statement

To many, mission statements are seen as examples of the discredited 'business' approach to health care produced by the White Paper (Department of Health, 1989). However, our own mission statement 'striving for the best in health care' is a surprisingly accurate encapsulation of our Trust's approach. We do strive — we are always on the look out for a better way — and we do unashamedly see the best as our goal.

## Core values

In 1994/5 the Trust set out to explicitly state its core values. From an initial working party the project was spread throughout the organization and eventually had direct participation from more than 1000 members of staff. As a result of this exercise we defined our core values as to:

- offer the best possible clinical care by sustaining staff skills and technology at the leading edge
- give patients the opportunity to play a real part in their own care
- ensure all staff exchange mutual respect and support
- deliver services in the way most convenient to patients
- provide an environment that promotes patients' comfort and wellbeing
- run the Trust in a way that empower staff to work effectively in the patients' interests
- protect each patient's right to courtesy, dignity, and their own spiritual and cultural needs.

## Developing excellence

The European Quality Foundation (Reed, 1998) model has been the engine of change in the Trust. Although predicated on achieving 'business excellence', it has been used increasingly in public service, where it has been found to be equally applicable.

## The commitment of key people

One consequence of becoming a Trust is the unequalled influence of the Chief Executive. Our Trust's Chief Executive has a strong commitment to quality in all aspects of the Trust's performance. His personal commitment has been allied to a devolved management style which involves key personnel, especially consultants, in the management process, and enables their own intrinsic drive for clinical excellence.

The Trust appears, therefore, to be extremely well placed culturally to respond to the challenge of clinical governance. However, there are some aspects of our performance which give cause for concern. These include the problem of quantity vs quality, equality of opportunity in the workforce, and research and development.

## Quality vs quantity

Over the last few years, the NHS has placed an enormous premium on quantity. In common with others, our Trust has responded by increasing workload at an inexorable rate. This has been at the expense of two aspects of quality. First, on occasions patient care has been less good than we would wish. Rushed consultations and overstretched nurses have been too frequent features of our work.

Second, there has been an enormous pressure on the staff — too many members of all professions are working too hard for too long. The pressures have been significantly exacerbated by the tendency of the centre to give inadequate time for responses to important questions. The feeling that our political and civil service masters are either out of touch with, or oblivious to, the destructive effects of their actions is having an alienating effect on staff and a corrosive effect on morale.

## Inequality of opportunity

Many aspects of professional development are well supported in our Trust, but the gap between the 'study leave' opportunities of doctors and nurses, for example, is wide and is a source of discontent.

## Research and development

For a Trust of our size and span, our research and development output is smaller than it should be. This partly reflects a relatively late development from a district general hospital (DGH) to a fully fledged tertiary centre, and partly the inexorable pressure of our clinical workload. There is increasing student teaching taking place in the Trust which we know, from feedback and external appraisal, is of very high quality, but the inequities of the service increment for teaching (SIFT) means that the rewards are meagre and the main resource is, yet again, extra work provided by already overburdened staff.

On balance we have concluded that our culture prepares us well for clinical governance, but there are significant areas in which we must improve.

## Do we have the right structure?

We examined our structures in two ways, first the management structure of the Trust, and second by examining the list of characteristics of a quality organization contained in the *White Paper The New NHS: Modern. Dependable* (Department of Health, 1997).

### Management structures

When the Trust was formed there was a wide-ranging debate regarding its future structure. It was agreed that the management should be based around individual patient teams. The result was 34 clinical directorates, either revolving round individual diagnostic groups, such as rheumatology, or individual patient groups, such as paediatrics. Each of these is managed by a consultant acting as clinical director and a clinical manager, who is usually, although not exclusively, a nurse.

In order to give each a voice on the management group the directorates are aggregated into divisions, each led by a consultant who is chief of service supported by a divisional manager — these people have diverse clinical and non-clinical backgrounds. The management group comprises the nine chiefs of service plus the corporate directors of the trust.

There are two important factors concerning this structure. First, there is a majority of doctors on the management group. Second, although the structure looks similar to that of many trusts which have clinical directors with equivalent spans to our chiefs, and sub-directors or lead clinicians where we have clinical directors, there are significant differences between these structures. Our own gives a high degree of autonomy to the directorates and a powerful clinical involvement, both medical and non-medical, in the directorate teams. Every directorate has budgetary responsibility, produces its own business plans and manages its own operation. This equates well to the statement in the White Paper:

> *'It is important that these arrangements for Clinical Governance engage professionals at ward and clinical level.'*

It is central to our concept of clinical governance that it will succeed, or fail, at this clinical level and it is our belief, based on the track record of our directorates, that they will be equal to, and managerially equipped for, the challenge.

## Characteristics of a quality organization

The White Paper listed the characteristics which are considered essential to ensure clinical quality. We evaluated the structures which we have in place to meet these criteria, using the matrix produced by the British Association of Medical Managers (BAMM, 1998). The first phase of the evaluation was to ask the chiefs (n=9) and clinical directors (n=18) in which areas they perceived our current practices to be robust. The result is shown in *Table 4.1*.

**Table 4.1: Quality audit: a checklist for clinical governance**

| System | Process established | Process explicit within organization | Process amenable to monitoring? | Reporting arrangements? | Implementation of findings/lessons monitored? | Levers & sanctions in place to make it work? |
|---|---|---|---|---|---|---|
| Adverse events detected investigated, lessons learnt translated into change in practice | ***** | **** | *** | *** | ** | * |
| Systematic learning from clinical complaints, with translation into change in practice | **** | *** | ** | * | * | ** |
| Poor clinical performance identified early and dealt with, skill, and speed and sensitivity, to avoid harm to patients | ** | * | * | * | 0 | 0 |
| Continuing professional development programmes in place reflecting principles of clinical governance | *** | ** | * | * | 0 | 0 |
| Quality of data for monitoring clinical care of consistently high standard | ** | * | * | 0 | 0 | 0 |
| Quality improvement process (clinical audit) intergrated into organizational quality programme | **** | *** | ** | * | * | 0 |
| Leadership skills developed at clinical team level | **** | ** | ** | 0 | 0 | 0 |
| Evidence-based practice and infrastructure in place and used | *** | ** | * | * | 0 | 0 |
| Clinical risk reduction programmes in place and of high quality | *** | ** | ** | * | * | 0 |

Medical managers' responses to question 'Do we have robust systems in place?' ***** = 100%, **** =75%, *** = 50%, ** =25%+; * = <25%, 0=0   Number of repondents: Chiefs n=9; Clinical directors n=18

There are several important messages in this. Obviously we have systems in place for all these aspects of the service, although the extent to which they might be considered 'robust' varies. Equally obvious is the diminishing confidence as the right-hand side of the matrix is approached — we are less good at explicit monitoring and reporting, and our levers and sanctions appear to be very weak.

Two areas produced particular anxieties. There was a high degree of dissatisfaction with our information services. These are less well developed than in some trusts, but further analysis showed that questions of definitions, varying interpretation by different parts of the service, and the inappropriate use of figures of dubious relevance and accuracy in such politically-motivated arenas as 'league tables' were greater causes of concern than our own in-house shortcomings. The ability to detect and deal with significant deficiencies in clinical performance was also a source of anxiety.

Our conclusion was that our organization did contain all the necessary attributes of a quality service, but that there were significant needs for strengthening them all and coordinating them better. One early role of the clinical governance committee will be to oversee these developments.

## What have we done?

Our stocktaking has led us to a series of actions designed to capitalize on our strengths and address our weaknesses. It was considered important that the medical director should lead the clinical governance process in the Trust and chair the clinical governance committee. The greatest strength of the Trust was felt to be its clinically led management structure, and it was agreed that this must be the fundamental building block on which all clinical governance activity should be built. Further analysis of our strengths and weaknesses is being undertaken, with, for example, all consultants being asked for their view through filling in the BAMM matrix; and more than 90% have done so.

Nurses and professions allied to medicine are being involved at all levels of the organization, but with encouragement to deliver through the directorate teams. There has been wide debate throughout the organization, and communication has been enhanced by production of a clinical governance newsletter and by setting up an intranet site. Because of the importance of lifelong learning, an associate medical director with specific responsibility for that area has been appointed. A guide to practical implementation of clinical governance for directorates has been developed containing a set of questions enabling directorates to benchmark themselves and plan their own development in an appropriate way.

## Are there lessons for others?

This chapter has described a single acute trust's initial response to the challenges posed by clinical governance. Others will recognize some aspects of their own organization, but none will be identical. Are there any messages for everyone? I believe there are four.

### Look critically at what you do now

There is more than one way of delivering clinical governance. Each organization must base its response on an honest analysis of its own style, strengths and weaknesses, and develop from there.

## Bed clinical governance into day-to-day management

If clinical governance becomes some sort of parallel universe detached from day-to-day management and practice, it is likely to produce a resented bureaucracy that fails to deliver. It is only by embedding its principles and practice into everyday care delivery and organization that it will succeed.

## Involve everyone

Management and professional divides, squabbling between professions and internecine professional disputes have all occurred and are all counter-productive — we are all in this together!

## Provide the right culture

There is an understandable tendency to concentrate on the mechanisms needed to deliver individual aspects of clinical governance. It is also likely that organizations such as the Commission for Health Improvement (CHIMP) will concentrate in this way. Some influential organizations are promoting their own methodologies, firmly based on a tick-box mind-set. For clinical governance to raise standards in a genuine and lasting fashion it must be developed in a supportive, blame-minimizing, educational atmosphere. The politicians' delight in 'name and shame' must not be allowed to flourish at the expense of creating a truly supportive, high quality, clinically driven organization.

---

**Key points**

The introduction of clinical governance should be based on:

- A structured analysis of present strengths and weaknesses

- Embedding it into everyday management and clinical structures

- Involving everyone in a supportive fashion

- Concentrating on providing the right atmosphere in which excellence can flourish, rather than simply developing mechanisms.

---

## References

British Association of Medical Managers (1998) *Clinical Governance in the New NHS.* British Association of Medical Managers, Cheadle, Cheshire

Department of Health (1989) *Working for Patients.* HMSO, London

Department of Health (1997) *The New NHS: Modern. Dependable.* Cmd 3807. HMSO, London

Department of Health (1998) *A First Class Service. Quality in the New NHS.* HMSO, London

Reed D (1998) *Central Government: Interpretation of the Business Excellence Model.* British Quality Foundation, London

# 6
# Clinical governance in primary care

*Stewart Drage*

Clinical governance is not new. In the same way that the Royal College of General Practitioners term 'primary care', invented in the 1950s, was only discovered by NHS management in the late 1980s, so clinical governance — or its component parts — has been with us far longer than management would have the non-medical public believe.

## The quality agenda

The term clinical governance first appeared in the white paper The New NHS, Modern Dependable (Department of Health, 1997) in December 1997, shortly after the general election. In its document *A First Class Service*, the government defined the term for the first time as:

> *'A framework through which NHS organisations are accountable for continuously improving the quality of their services and safeguarding high standards of care by creating an environment in which excellence in clinical care will flourish.'* (Department of Health, 1998)

The government was driven by the need to restore confidence in the NHS, especially after the cardiac surgery inquiry in Bristol, as well as the need to deliver a higher quality service across the country, and be seen to do so in its first term.

Essentially, the government was announcing to the profession that it wished to see greater accountability to the public for clinical decisions, and that a regulatory framework would be established across the NHS to see that this was done.

## How will clinical governance operate?

The framework rests on four pillars, which are now part of British law following the Royal Assent of the Health Act 1999 on June 30. These are:

### A duty of quality

Every practitioner and organization within the NHS now has a statutory duty to ensure that they strive to provide the highest quality of care. GPs and their practices are now accountable to their primary care group (PCG) boards (through the clinical governance lead member — the primary care equivalent to clinical director), and PCGs are in turn accountable to health authorities. The chief executive of the health authority is accountable direct to parliament, and therefore has a strong interest in ensuring that the clinical governance framework is firmly bedded in.

### NICE

The National Institute for Clinical Excellence has been established to 'even out' differences across the country by pronouncing on the plethora of guidelines, and on controversial issues such as the use of interferon B.

## CHImp

The Commission for Health Improvement (CHImp) has the powers to carry out investigations in GP practices, PCGs and trusts, to determine whether or not there is or has been unsatisfactory practice.

### Self-regulation

The government has enhanced the powers of local medical committees and has invited the General Medical Council (GMC) to submit proposals for more rigorous sanctions for aberrant doctors.

# What is happening right now?

In the meantime, across the UK, and differently in each of the four countries, GPs, nurses, local authorities and the public have been learning about working together in the spirit of partnership set out in the new NHS. Clinical governance has naturally been high on their list of priorities, but until now most PCGs have been too concerned with establishing their own internal structures and with understanding how to make their new budgetary arrangements work.

This is somewhat fortuitous as the Health Act 1999 had not yet appeared, very little guidance had been forthcoming from the NHS Executive on how to implement clinical governance, and very few authors had yet produced anything concrete for general consumption. However, PCGs are beginning to get on top of these affairs, and are now turning their attention to the detail of clinical governance. They are examining how to make it effective, yet retain the confidence of individual practitioners.

Pulling this off will be tricky. GP and nurse morale continues to remain low, while cynicism about resources is high. *A First Class Service* (1998) goes to great lengths to reassure practitioners that clinical governance is about the pursuit of excellence, and not about naming and shaming, yet the media continue to pander unabated to the public's apparent desire for the latter. It will be a very special PCG board which can successfully manage that triangle.

Most boards are approaching the challenge by acknowledging that most of the fabric of clinical governance already exists, and that good governance can be demonstrated by highlighting the building blocks, resourcing them, making them more widely available so that they reach out to all, and then focusing down on one or two priorities which fit with the PCG's needs in terms of their Health Improvement Programme (HimP), prescribing, or other areas of interest/concern. The building blocks available to them are:

## Clinical audit

Medical audit advisory groups (MAAGs), or similar, have been firmly established across the country for over 10 years. Funded on a shoestring by Family Practitioner Committees (FPCs), Family Health Services Authorities (FHSAs) and subsequently health authorities, they have been treated with enthusiasm by the vast majority of GPs. Organized by GPs for GPs, they have positively facilitated audit within practices and demonstrate that there is a firm base for clinical audit within primary care.

Two key adjustments will need to happen if MAAGs or their successors are to fit in with the new NHS. First they will need to be more inclusive and involve other primary care health professionals, especially nurses, and second they will need to coordinate audit work and focus on the priorities of the PCG, and not the preferences of the individual GP — in other words, they must become service orientated as opposed to academically orientated.

## Continuing professional development

Current education and training arrangements will also need to adapt, if they are to meet the service-linked requirements of the new NHS. Continuing medical education, until now for most GPs a non-directed exercise incentivised through the postgraduate education allowance, will become more directed and will incorporate service-based training — an element which has long been the Cinderella of the NHS, and for post vocational training scheme GPs practically non-existent.

Training will need to reflect both the needs of the doctor and the demands of the service. It will also increasingly need to be seen to be coordinated in a multidisciplinary fashion. If it is to succeed, this new approach will need to command the confidence of GPs. Care will be needed to ensure that existing good practice is not sacrificed in pursuit of unachievable perfection. Service-based education and training requires substantial investment by the service in the protected learning time for its participants. The track record of the NHS in this field is appalling.

## Research and development

NHS Executive investment in research and development in primary care is growing, and will require ongoing resourcing if it is to deliver solutions to the many dilemmas facing a service confronting the need to minimize waiting lists and length of hospital stays.

## Clinical risk management

No clinical management plan is without risk: health outcome risk for patients, and medicolegal risk for practitioners. In general practice, GPs as independent contractors are not protected by a trust or health authority from medicolegal risk. As the traditionally low-risk nature of primary care becomes more complex, so too does the level and variety of that risk. The new quality-led, cash-limited NHS can no longer tolerate avoidable errors, and needs to minimize the impact of unavoidable errors.

For some disease processes, protocols and guidelines, when adequately evaluated, may go some way to lowering risk, but the generalist nature of British general practice does not readily lend itself to the protocol approach, and is itself at risk if such an approach is too rigorously or too innocently pursued. Much more research needs to be urgently done in this field. GPs and patients will need to come to terms with a potential loss of some of the arguably softer psycho-social aspects of a visit to the surgery — so often an integral part of continuity of care so unique to British general practice and the envy of most other nations — in pursuit of a more outpatient styled and purist medical model of consultation.

## Poor performance

In 1996, legislation enabled the GMC to institute proceedings in cases of poorly performing doctors. Serious cases which cause a GP's registration to be in question are dealt with through the GMC's performance procedures. The GMC advises that other cases are normally resolved locally in accordance with the School of Health and Related Research (SCHARR) report (Rotherham et al, 1997) aimed at identifying underlying causes and proposing remedies. Clinical governance at PCG level provides a mechanism for such local resolution to take place at an earlier stage, freeing up the local SCHARR procedures to manage the more complex cases.

## The complaints procedures

The Wilson report (Department of Health, 1994) led to a radical revision of the NHS complaints procedures. Separation of investigation from discipline has resulted in successful local resolution of the vast majority of complaints at practice level, with very few cases ending up at independent review. As part of clinical governance, data from the complaints process will provide a useful adjunct to the enhancement of quality and risk management.

## Applying clinical governance in primary care

In practical terms, PCG clinical governance lead members have now been appointed. Their role is to ensure that processes exist within practices for GPs and nurses to meet their duty of quality obligations, to determine what resources might be needed to operate those arrangements, and to begin to identify areas of concern which might need addressing.

As a start, they will encourage GPs and nurses to ensure that the education and training in which they participate is relevant to their needs, and to focus on one or two areas which are priorities for the PCG, such as diabetes management and prescribing costs. With the very limited resources available to them, these should fully occupy their time in the first year. The more enthusiastic PCGs will attempt to deal with a wider range of issues, but will need to maintain the confidence of their GPs and nurses as they progress their agenda.

PCG boards will be looking to their clinical governance leads and support staff to ensure constant improvement in their organizations' clinical quality, prescribing practices and budgetary control. They will increasingly use financial levers to encourage compliance with the PCG's needs, and they will be performance-managed on their results.

## Next steps

Primary Care Trust status — thought by many to be the precursors of American-style Health Maintenance Organizations in Britain — will certainly depend on the demonstration of good clinical governance, and there will therefore be some considerable variation in the style and nature of clinical governance delivery, depending on how much the PCG covets trust status. But if the experience of the previous NHS reforms is anything to go by, we can expect widescale Primary Care Trust status to be achieved sooner rather than later. We will then be able to assess the impact of clinical governance if not in terms of outcomes for patients, then certainly in terms of the structure of the service, well ahead of the government's original 10-year agenda.

Whether primary care will be any better at meeting patients' expectations remains to be seen.

### Key points

- Clinical governance seeks to make clinical decision-making accountable to the public.

- There is a new duty of quality on all working in the NHS.

- Many elements of clinical governance already flourish in practice.

- Attention should be paid to developing systems to manage clinical risk.

- A bottom-up approach to clinical governance is more likely to succeed.

## References

Department of Health (1994) *Being Heard. The report of a review committee on NHS complaints procedures.* HMSO, London

Department of Health (1997) *The New NHS Modern, Dependable.* HMSO, London

Department of Health (1998) *A First Class Service.* HMSO, London

Rotherham G, Martin D, Joesbury H, Mathers N (1997) *Measure to Assist GPs whose Performance Gives Cause for Concern.* School of Health and Related Research at the University of Sheffield, Sheffield

# 7
# Clinical governance and revalidation

*Hilary Thomas*

The climate change has been underway for some time: the publication in 1995 of the General Medical Council (GMC)'s Good Medical Practice, with its explicit standards of good care, showed that the profession recognized the demands for quality assurance and partnership. The GMC's Performance Procedures were another step in that direction. Events such as the Bristol case at the GMC, and subsequent government enquiry have added impetus to the process (Irvine, 1997a,b).

The government is ensuring that the momentum is maintained through the establishment of bodies such as the National Institute for Clinical Effectiveness (NICE) and the Commission for Health Improvement. For the medical profession, and the guardian of its register — the GMC, we cannot afford to remain recumbent and reactive. We too must roll up our sleeves and put our house in order.

We may well feel that the vast majority of doctors are already delivering a good standard of care, and that it is unfair to lumber them with the blame for a small minority of poor performers. However, it is clear that our traditional system of exception reporting is not sufficient, and has failed patients in a number of high-profile examples: we cannot expect to qualify and sit happily on the medical register for the next 30 years as long as no misdemeanour has come to light.

In February 1999 the GMC made the decision that all doctors should be 'up-to-date' and 'fit to practise'. The ability to demonstrate those two assets of any practising doctor would then be linked to their remaining on the medical register.

It is the quality of the NHS as a whole on which we must now focus, not simply the management of poorly performing doctors (Chantler, 1999; Irvine, 1999). The objective must be to raise the overall standard. There will still be a small minority beyond the pale and it is through the fitness to practise procedures of the GMC that their registration will be restricted or removed. But revalidation is about the achievements, and the continuous improvement, of those doctors remaining on the register (more than 100,000 in active practice), and the GMC has already agreed that revalidation will be based on its document *Good Medical Practice*.

## Relationship between clinical governance and revalidation

There are four components of clinical governance:

1. The creation of clear lines of accountability for the over-all quality of clinical care

2. A comprehensive programme of quality improvement activities'. These might include the participation of docors in audit, national confidential inquiries, support for and use of evidence-based practice, and implementation of both national service framework and NICE recommendations

3. Systems to assess and reduce clinical risk should be in place

4.  All professional groups should identify and remedy poor performance.

This may entail the reporting of adverse incidents so that lessons can be learnt before the situation is irredeemable (Hopkinson, 1999). Many of the fundamental ingredients are common with those which will be required for the development and implementation of revalidation — audit, appraisal and a constructive approach to teamwork such as that needed to implement evidence.

## Where is the GMC at?

Currently it is reasonable to say that revalidation is in its developmental phase. There is a matrix of work to be undertaken, which entails a wide consultative process with extensive lay involvement at each stage both in the development and the implementation. The GMC is beginning to define the kinds of evidence which each doctor will need to produce in order to be revalidated.

While implementation per se may not be as important an issue for the GMC as development, it is important that the position at which the GMC arrives by May 2001 is consistent with local processes and capable of implementation: revalidation must not entail new bureaucratic systems, it should draw upon data generated under clinical governance. There is a very important exercise with hearts and minds so that the majority of the profession and the public are brought with the process — not dragged, kicking and screaming. On the ground the Oxford Local Medical Regulation Project is taking place in parallel, under the auspices of a group entitled Maintaining

Good Medical Practice. An external steering group includes the relevant players (Royal Colleges, UKCC, British Association of Medical Managers (BAMM), postgraduate deans, deans, Association of Community Health Councils of England and Wales).

The objective of the Oxford project is to ensure that there are good local systems in place for implementing the two documents *Good Medical Practice* and *Maintaining Good Medical Practice* (GMC, 1998). This will be possible by defining how those with responsibility for local systems could monitor the implementation of these documents. While the Oxford project is not about revalidation or clinical governance in its entirety, it is about interrogating the processes and ensuring that they are robust and fit for purpose.

The project is valid in its own right. But it has been developed at the same time as the discussions about revalidation have been taking place and the government has been establishing its quality framework. It aims to provide assistance to professional (medical) self-regulation. It may also contribute to the delivery of revalidation processes.

The Oxford project has taken a number of doctors as case studies — mapping the doctor's journey through the career pathway and asking a series of questions about the processes of appointment, development and departure as well as enquiring about remediation.

Much of what will be required by chief executives to demonstrate that clinical governance is being implemented within their own organizations will represent the component parts of the 'revalidation process'. It is very important that this process is not onerous and does not reinvent an entirely new tier of processes for those who cause concern.

The GMC is also tapping into other examples of good local medical regulation. Great Ormond Street has developed processes for appraisal, which were implemented from the medical director down — true management by walking about. The process to date has shown the paucity of public involvement in medical regulation at local level. This involvement will be more explicit than before by examining a matrix of factors involved in practice. The other important factor is not to alarm the public by seeking their involvement without their understanding of its importance. There is no doubt that public expectation has risen — the medical profession now needs to grasp the nettle and make it clear that they actively seek public involvement and hence public ownership of the result.

The Chief Medical Officers have been consulted as part of an attempt to be explicit, to ensure the involvement of the NHS and to check that there is no duplication or dissonance with other initiatives. Effective implementation will need both local and NHS Executive support. One clear message is that revalidation and clinical governance must not result in duplication but should mesh in such a way that Trusts and the individual doctors can achieve their objectives — bearing in mind that a high proportion of doctors on the medical register, particularly GPs, will not be involved in clinical governance.

I am enough of an optimist to believe that no competent, reasonable doctor should have anything to fear from revalidation. Indeed if the initial objectives set out are fulfilled we should all benefit, and have a medical workforce of which we can be justly proud. Much hard work is still to be done before we achieve that end, but the more we get our hands dirty at this stage the more likely we are to be able to live with the consequences. There is no mileage in carping from the sidelines — the world has moved on — openness, transparency and public accountability are here to stay. Better that we work in partnership with patients, management and others, using our professional ethics — to the benefit of patients, the public and the service we provide — than that we find ourselves imposed with an ugly chimaera of others' demands.

### Key points

- The new agenda for the NHS is quality.

- Revalidation and clinical governance are important components of that agenda and its delivery.

- Revalidation is about being 'up to date' and 'fit to practice'.

- Revalidation must be straightforward and implementable. It must not reinvent or duplicate existing frameworks but incorporate them.

- Revalidation should not be feared by the vast majority of doctors who are competent and reasonable.

## References

Chantler C (1999) The role and education of doctors in the delivery of health care. *Lancet* **353**: 1178–81

Department of Health (1998) *A First Class Service: Quality in the New NHS*. Health Circular HSC 1998/113. Department of Health, London

Department of Health (1999) *Clinical Governance: Quality in the New NHS*. Health Circular HSC 1999/065. Department of Health, London

General Medical Council (1995) *Good Medical Practice.* General Medical
     Council, London
Hopkinson RB (1999) Clinical governance: putting it into practice in an
     acute trust. *Clinician in Management* **8**: 81–8
Irvine D (1997a) The performance of doctors. 1: Professionalism and self
     regulation in a changing world. *Br Med J* **314**: 1540–2
Irvine D (1997b) The performance of doctors. II: Maintaining good
     practice, protecting patients from poor performance. *Br Med J* **314**:
     1613–15
Irvine D (1999) The performance of doctors: the new  professionalism.
     *Lancet* **353**: 1174–7

# 8
# Clinical governance: what it is, what it isn't and what it should be

*Ian Gilmore*

The term clinical governance has no rivals in its rate of rise from obscurity to top of the medical pops. Two years ago it 'appeared' as an extension of corporate governance, placing a statutory requirement on NHS trusts to put systems in place for ensuring quality of clinical care as well as for 'balancing their books' — meeting clinical as well as financial standards. However, it soon developed overtones of very much more.

These statutory obligations on trusts to ensure clinical as well as corporate governance are firmly the responsibility of the Chief Executive, putting him/her and not the clinicians at risk of imprisonment for failure to deliver. However, in practice it has been the clinician, particularly the hospital consultant, who has been the focus of early attention in the 'post-Bristol era', and while this is hardly surprising it is nonetheless unfortunate.

Clinical governance comes at a time when clinicians are feeling ever more vulnerable from rising workload pressures, from a diminishing service contribution by 'post-Calman' junior doctors and from an erosion of individual clinical freedom. When the discussions should have been primarily about systems, they have been hijacked by issues of individual performance — the poorly performing doctor. Add to this the emergence of the National Institute of Clinical Excellence (NICE) and the Commission for Health Improvement (CHI), the related issue of revalidation and the (entirely reasonable) attempts of the General Medical Council (GMC) and the Royal

Colleges to take the high ground and the scene is set for resigned confusion within the profession.

I can not claim any particular insight or wisdom, but I can look from two perspectives, that of (until 12 months ago) a Medical Director of a large, acute, University Trust and now an officer of a Royal Medical College (the Royal College of Physicians) in the thick of trying to establish national policies that make sense for the thousands of physicians doing their best to look after their patients.

## The components of clinical governance

The essential foundations are as follows:
- the setting of realistic and evidence-based standards of care
- the monitoring of performance against these standards
- the implementation of change to ensure that thest standards are reached and, if possible, exceeded.

The tools that are used in the achievement of these components are many, and include:
- multidisciplinary clinical audit
- clinical effectiveness
- research and development
- lifelong learning
- risk management and critical incident reporting
- evidence-based medicine
- guidelines, pathways and protocols
- service accreditation
- individual appraisal and assessment
- information management.

## Standard setting

In order to be credible, a standard has to be:
- Important to patients and their care
- Evidence based — there have to be strong grounds for believing that achievement of a standard brings about an improvement in the outcome of care
- generalizable — it has to apply to different parts of the NHS across the country
- achievable — if only 10% of units in the country have any chance of reaching a standard, it is not useful.

this end the standard has to be nationally-agreed. Some may come from National Service Frameworks and Health Improvement Programmes, but the Colleges and specialist societies are ideally placed to devise early and simple standards that the vast majority of clinicians would accept. It must be remembered that there is no point in selecting standards measurable only by an outcome that may be 10–20 years away. This may be appropriate for epidemiologists but it will hardly satisfy the public about the standard of their local hospital.

For this reason it may be necessary to use outcome-validated process measurements. For instance, the numbers of patients being discharged from hospital after myocardial infarction who are taking aspirin may be a reasonable surrogate marker for quality of care that reduces long-term mortality. Standards may be agreed statements of service requirements, such as the need for a minimum of two consultants in a specialty in order to maintain a service for 52 weeks per year.

Within the Royal College of Physicians, we are currently asking the 24 subspecialties for which we have responsibility to identify two or three standards that would meet the above criteria for a credible standard.

## Monitoring standards

As in setting of standards, achievability is crucial to the monitoring of them. There is no place for standards that cannot be measured with existing information systems and audit methods. Ideally the data should be captured during normal clinical activity such as clinic letters or discharge summaries.

### Monitoring the individual clinician

There are some areas where the individual clinician should be assessed rather than monitoring outcomes of units or services. For instance, each individual should be required to demonstrate that he or she is keeping up to date with their continuing medical education, and this can be checked at the time of the annual review of job plan, already a part of life in most trusts. This assessment should be linked to other obvious clinical governance issues like complaints, medicolegal actions and critical incident reports, but it must be a two-way review in which the clinician may highlight the barriers to improving care in his/her area (such as equipment and other resource deficiencies).

## Monitoring the service

This is an attractive alternative to the above, because there are great concerns about the feasibility of assessing the performance of individual clinicians over a wide range of skills and competencies.

The detailed assessment of clinical skills undertaken by the GMC when a clinician's competence is called into question is simply impossible to implement as a tool to regularly monitor the performance of all practising doctors. However, it may be feasible to examine the performance of a unit or service, with the assumption that if that unit is achieving high scores for competence then the constituent parts, the individual clinicians, are performing well. If a unit or service fails such an assessment then the individual components would require closer scrutiny. This 'peer service review' has been piloted in several medical specialties, particularly in chest medicine by the British Thoracic Society. It has a valuable 'buddying' or mentoring function and the visitors as well as the visited benefit from the exchange of ideas, but it will have to develop a tougher, pass-fail mentality to satisfy managers and politicians in the post-Bristol wake.

Furthermore, the practicality of yet another round of visits, on top of those of the postgraduate deans, the College visits for senior house officer and specialist registrar posts, the task force and the GMC, to name but a few, raises the spectre of everyone's time and energies being expended in visiting and being visited to the detriment of clinical service. The best opportunity would seem to be to roll up together some of these varied activities. However, we desperately need evidence that they work.

# Implementation of change

The setting and monitoring of standards outlined is of little value unless the 'loop can be closed' by correcting identified deficiencies.

## Resource deficiencies

This is where clinical governance can and should be to the advantage of the competent and conscientious clinician. First, he/she is obliged to demonstrate that existing resources are being used as effectively as possible, and quite rightly managers no longer respond immediately to 'shroud-waving'. Nonetheless the vast majority of problems in service provision are because of woefully deficient investment in them. The solutions must be innovative, cost-effective and bring about improved care for patients.

## The poorly-performing doctor

This is where the spotlight of clinical governance has been, although the vast majority of hospital doctors work very hard to keep up to date and to deliver a high quality of service. Of course we must take some responsibility for that spotlight, because as a profession we have failed to deal with the small minority who have not lived up to reasonable standards. This is occasionally a straightforward problem of incompetence but is much more often a complex mixture of conduct, personality and performance issues. It is usually not difficult to identify these colleagues, but the problem in the past has been what to do about them.

This has been starkly clarified by the GMC, and no doctor should now be in any doubt about his/her professional responsibility to draw to the employer's attention, usually through the medical director, any concerns about the competence of colleagues. The next step is now the difficult one, and the medical director has to decide if patients are at immediate risk (in which case the doctor must be suspended pending further investigation). He/she must initiate an appropriate investigation and then decide whether the individual's registration should be called into question (in which case the GMC should be informed) or if local resolution is possible. The medical director has a heavy responsibility, but common sense goes a long way in helping to decide the best course of action.

## The role of the UK Medical Royal Colleges

While clinical governance is primarily the responsibility of individual NHS providers, the Royal Colleges are uniquely placed to assist. Their core function is the maintenance and improvement of clinical standards, and they are by and large respected for their independence by both the NHS and individual doctors. They provide the following potential opportunities:

1. Setting nationally agreed, appropriate clinical standards, in conjunction with other national bodies

2. Monitoring performance against these standards by developing achievable national frameworks for clinical audit

3 Assisting trusts in annual appraisal and assessment programmes through their network of regional and local advisers

4. Arranging continuing medical education and coninuing professional development programmes and monitoring the participation and achievement of clincians in these programmes

5. Arranging multidisciplinary external service reiews from time to time

6. Assisting trusts by sending in a team of indeendent advisers where there are concerns about the outcomes or performance within a clinical unit

7. Assisting trusts in the mentoring process and arranging retraining if appropriate for individual doctors identified as having difficulties before patients are put at risk.

The case for reviewing doctors' right to practice from time to time through revalidating their registration with the GMC is a powerful one, and the building blocks for this should be the demonstration of success in steps 1–5 above.

## Conclusions

Clinical governance has as many opportunities as threats, and it is only through early, active and explicit involvement that clinicians can protect themselves from unwarranted slurs as well as improving the care of their patients.

### Key points

- The emphasis of clinical governance should be on ensuring that systems are in place to help clinicians provide high quality care.

- Doctors must take the lead in setting evidence-based, achievable standards that can be monitored in their specialty.

- Medical Royal Colleges, working with specialist societies, are best placed to put together the framework to support clinicians and to allow them to demonstrate their continuing fitness to practice.

## References

NHS Executive (1998) *A First Class Service. Quality in the New NHS.* NHS Executive, Leeds

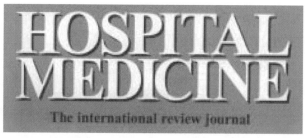

Hospital Medicine is an international, peer-reviewed clinical review journal. It covers all hospital specialties, as reflected by its Editorial Board and International Advisory Board. It contains review articles written by experts in each field, allowing busy doctors to quickly and easily update their knowledge on a particular area. It was launched in 1966 and since then has constantly provided doctors with an independent source of clinical information in an easily digestible format.

## Each issue contains:

- Editorials
- One symposium containing 3/4 articles on 1 topic. The subject of each symposium will be led by speciality.
- Review articles
- Case reports
- Management article
- Education and training update - two articles each issue looking at issues affecting both trainers and trainees
- Correspondence
- Book reviews

**To order your copy of
Hospital Medicine,
please call 0800 137 201**

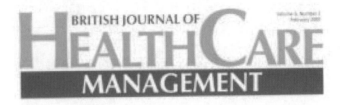

BRITISH JOURNAL OF HEALTHCARE MANAGEMENT

British Journal of Health Care Management has recently seen a fresh new design and continues to offer you the best opportunity to keep one step ahead. The journal's broad ranging review articles and topical and intelligent analysis gives it an authority and cutting edge that cannot be found elsewhere.

**Each issue contains:**

- Editorials
- Comment
- Policy developments
- Andrew Roth's Westminster
- Inside information
- Talking point
- Book reviews
- Management reviews
- Bosanquet's view
- Alan Maynard
- Supplements

**To order your copy of
British Journal of Health Care Management
please call 0800 137 201**

**04426399**